Ketogenic Diet Lunch & Dinner Cookbook

Delightful, Budget-Friendly and Simple Recipes for a Slimmer You

Justice Craft

CONTENTS

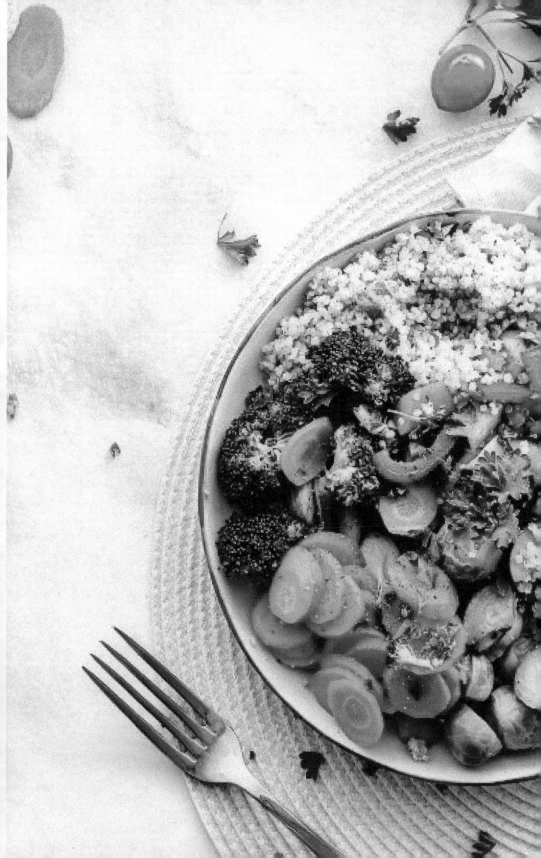

Pesto Zoodles

Ingredients for 4 servings

2/3 cup grated Pecorino Romano cheese

2 tbsp olive oil

1 white onion, chopped

1 garlic clove, minced

28 oz tofu, pressed and cubed

1 red bell pepper, sliced

6 zucchinis, spiralized

Salt and black pepper to taste

¼ cup basil pesto

½ cup shredded mozzarella

Toasted pine nuts to garnish

Instructions - Total Time: around 20 minutes

Heat olive oil in a pot and sauté onion and garlic for 3 minutes. Add in tofu

and cook until golden on all sides, then pour in the

bell pepper and cook for 4

minutes. Mix in zucchini, pour pesto on top, and season with salt and pepper.

Cook for 3-4 minutes. Stir in the Pecorino cheese. Top with mozzarella,

garnish with pine nuts, and serve.

Per serving: Cal 477; Net Carbs 5.4g; Fat 32g; Protein 20g

Caprese Casserole

Ingredients for 4 servings

1 cup mozzarella cheese, cubed

1 cup cherry tomatoes, halved

2 tbsp basil pesto

1 cup mayonnaise

2 oz Parmesan cheese

1 cup arugula

4 tbsp olive oil

Instructions - Total Time: around 25 minutes

Preheat oven to 350 F. In a baking dish, mix cherry tomatoes, mozzarella

cheese, basil pesto, mayonnaise, and half of the Parmesan cheese. Level the

ingredients with a spatula and sprinkle the remaining Parmesan cheese on

top. Bake for 20 minutes until the top is golden brown; let cool. Slice, top with arugula and olive oil, and serve.

Per serving: Cal 450; Net Carbs 5g; Fat 41g; Protein 12g

Veal Chops with Raspberry Sauce

Ingredients for 4 servings

3 tbsp olive oil

2 lb veal chops

Salt and black pepper to taste

2 cups raspberries

¼ cup water

1 ½ tbsp Italian Herb mix

3 tbsp balsamic vinegar

2 tsp Worcestershire sauce

Instructions - Total Time: around 20 minutes

Heat oil in a skillet over medium heat, season veal with salt and pepper, and

cook for 5 minutes on each side. Put on serving plates and reserve the veal

drippings. Mash the raspberries in a bowl until jam-like. Pour into a

saucepan, add water, and herb mix. Bring to boil on

low heat for 4 minutes.

Stir in veal drippings, balsamic vinegar, and Worcestershire sauce. Simmer

for 1 minute. Spoon sauce over the veal chops and serve.

Per serving: Cal 413; Net Carbs 1.1g; Fat 32g; Protein 26g

Cheddar Quesadillas with Leafy Greens

Ingredients for 4 servings

3 eggs

½ cup cream cheese

1½ tsp psyllium husk powder

1 tbsp coconut flour

½ tsp salt

1 tbsp butter, softened

5 oz grated cheddar cheese

1 oz leafy greens

Instructions - Total Time: around 30 minutes

Preheat oven to 400 F. In a bowl, whisk the eggs with cream cheese. In

another bowl, combine psyllium husk, coconut flour, and salt. Add in the egg

mixture and mix until fully incorporated. Let sit for a few minutes. Line a baking sheet with parchment paper and pour in half of the mixture. Bake the

tortilla for 7 minutes until brown around the edges. Repeat with the

remaining batter. Grease a skillet with the butter and place in a tortilla.

Sprinkle with cheddar cheese, leafy greens and cover with another tortilla.

Brown each side for 1 minute. Serve.

Per serving: Cal 470; Net Carbs 4g; Fat 40g; Protein 19g

Curried Tofu with Buttery Cabbage

Ingredients for 4 servings

2 cups extra firm tofu, cubed

2 tbsp coconut oil

½ cup grated coconut

1 tsp yellow curry powder

½ tsp onion powder

2 cups Napa cabbage

4 oz butter

Lemon wedges for serving

Instructions - Total Time: around 55 minutes

In a bowl, mix grated coconut, curry powder, salt, and onion powder. Toss in

tofu. Heat coconut oil in a skillet and fry tofu until golden brown; transfer to

a plate. In the same skillet, melt half of butter and sauté the cabbage until slightly caramelized. Place the cabbage into plates with tofu and lemon

wedges. Melt the remaining butter in the skillet and drizzle over the cabbage

and tofu. Serve.

Per serving: Cal 733; Net Carbs 4g; Fat 61g; Protein 36g

BBQ Pork Skewers with Squash Mash

Ingredients for 4 servings

7 tbsp fresh cilantro, chopped

4 tbsp fresh basil, chopped

2 garlic cloves

Juice of ½ a lemon

4 tbsp capers

2/3 cup olive oil

Salt and black pepper to taste

1 lb pork tenderloin, cubed

½ tbsp sugar-free BBQ sauce

½ cup butter

3 cups butternut squash, cubed

2 oz grated Parmesan

Instructions - Total Time: around 30 minutes

In a blender, add cilantro, basil, garlic, lemon juice,

capers, olive oil, salt, and

pepper and process until smooth. Set aside the salsa verde. Thread pork cubes

on skewers. Season with salt and brush with BBQ sauce.

Melt 1 tbsp butter in a grill pan and sear the skewers until browned on both

sides; remove to a plate. Pour squash into a pot, add some salted water, and

bring to a boil for 15 minutes. Drain and pour the squash into a bowl. Add in

the remaining butter, Parmesan cheese, salt, and pepper and mash everything.

Serve the skewers with mashed squash and salsa verde.

Per serving: Cal 850; Net Carbs 5g; Fat 78g; Protein 26g

Buttered Carrot Noodles with Kale

Ingredients for 4 servings

2 carrots, spiralized

¼ cup vegetable broth

4 tbsp butter

1 garlic clove, minced

1 cup chopped kale

Salt and black pepper to serve

Instructions - Total Time: around 15 minutes

Pour broth into a saucepan over low heat and add in carrot noodles to simmer

for 3 minutes; strain and set aside. Melt butter in a skillet and sauté garlic and

kale until the kale is wilted. Pour in carrots, season with salt and pepper, and

stir-fry for 4 minutes. Serve with grilled pork.

Per serving: Cal 335; Net Carbs 8g; Fat 28g; Protein

6g

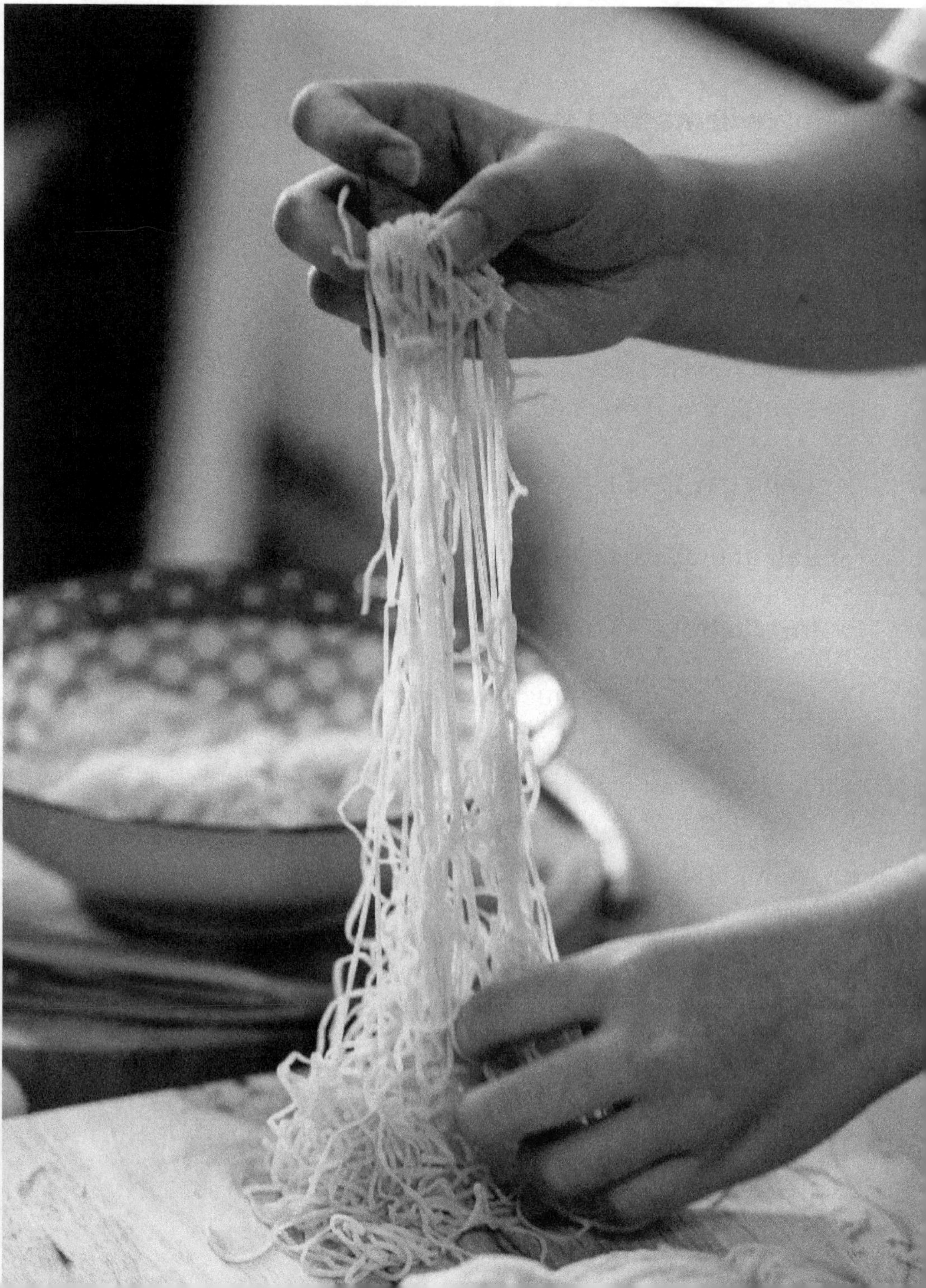

Spicy Veggie Steaks with Green Salad

Ingredients for 2 servings

⅓ eggplant, sliced

½ zucchini, sliced

¼ cup coconut oil

Juice of ½ lemon

5 oz cheddar cheese, cubed

10 Kalamata olives

2 tbsp pecans

1 oz mixed salad greens

½ cup mayonnaise

½ tsp Cayenne pepper

Instructions - Total Time: around 35 minutes

Set the oven to broil and line a baking sheet with parchment paper. Arrange

zucchini and eggplant slices on the sheet. Brush with

coconut oil and sprinkle

with cayenne pepper. Broil until golden brown, about 18 minutes. Remove to

a serving platter and drizzle with lemon juice. Arrange cheddar cheese,

olives, pecans, and mixed greens next to grilled veggies. Top with

mayonnaise and serve.

Per serving: Cal 512g; Net Carbs 8g; Fat 31g; Protein 22g

Tofu & Bok Choy Stir-Fry

Ingredients for 4 servings

2 ½ cups baby bok choy, quartered lengthwise

5 oz butter

2 cups extra firm tofu, cubed

Salt and black pepper to taste

1 tsp garlic powder

1 tsp onion powder

1 tbsp plain vinegar

2 garlic cloves, minced

1 tsp chili flakes

1 tbsp fresh ginger, grated

3 green onions, sliced

Instructions - Total Time: around 45 minutes

Melt half of butter in a wok over medium heat, add bok choy, and stir-fry

until softened. Season with salt, pepper, garlic and

onion powders, and plain

vinegar. Sauté for 2 minutes and set aside. Melt the remaining butter in the

wok and sauté garlic, chili flakes, and ginger until fragrant. Put in tofu and

cook until browned. Add in green onions and bok choy and cook for 2

minutes. Serve warme.

Per serving: Cal 686; Net Carbs 8g; Fat 64g; Protein 35g

Avocado Coconut Pie

Ingredients for 4 servings

1 egg

4 tbsp coconut flour

4 tbsp chia seeds

¾ cup almond flour

1 tbsp psyllium husk powder

1 tsp baking powder

3 tbsp coconut oil

2 ripe avocados, chopped

1 cup mayonnaise

2 tbsp fresh parsley, chopped

1 jalapeño pepper, chopped

½ tsp onion powder

½ cup cream cheese

1¼ cups grated Parmesan

Instructions - Total Time: around 80 minutes

Preheat oven to 350 F. In a food processor, add coconut flour, chia seeds,

almond flour, psyllium husk, baking powder, coconut oil, and 4 tbsp water.

Blend until the resulting dough forms into a ball.

Line a springform pan with parchment paper and spread the dough. Bake for

15 minutes. In a bowl, put avocado, mayonnaise, egg, parsley, jalapeño

pepper, onion powder, cream cheese, and Parmesan cheese; mix well.

Remove the piecrust when ready and fill with the creamy mixture. Bake for

35 minutes until lightly golden brown.

Per serving: Cal 876; Net Carbs 10g; Fat 67g; Protein 24g

Beef Cakes with Broccoli Mash

Ingredients for 4 servings

1 egg

1 lb ground beef

½ white onion, chopped

2 tbsp olive oil

1 lb broccoli

5 tbsp butter, softened

2 oz grated Parmesan

2 tbsp lemon juice

Instructions - Total Time: around 30 minutes

In a bowl, add ground beef, egg, onion, salt, and pepper. Mix and mold out 6-

8 cakes out of the mixture. Warm olive oil in a skillet and fry the patties for

6-8 minutes on both sides. Remove to a plate.

Pour lightly salted water into a pot over medium heat, bring to a boil, and add broccoli. Cook until tender but not too soft, 6-8 minutes. Drain and transfer to

a bowl. Add in 2 tbsp of butter, and Parmesan cheese. Use an immersion

blender to puree the ingredients until smooth and creamy; set aside. To make

the lemon butter, mix remaining butter with lemon juice, salt, and pepper in a

bowl. Serve the cakes with broccoli mash and lemon butter.

Per serving: Cal 860; Net Carbs 6g; Fat 76g; Protein 35g

Baked Cheesy Spaghetti Squash

Ingredients for 4 servings

2 lb spaghetti squash

1 tbsp coconut oil

Salt and black pepper to taste

2 tbsp melted butter

½ tbsp garlic powder

1/5 tsp chili powder

1 cup coconut cream

2 oz cream cheese

1 cup grated mozzarella

2 oz grated Parmesan

2 tbsp fresh cilantro, chopped

Instructions - Total Time: around 40 minutes

Preheat oven to 350 F. Cut squash in halves lengthwise and spoon out the

seeds and fiber. Place the halves on a baking dish,

brush each with coconut

oil and season with salt and pepper. Bake for 30 minutes. Remove and use

two forks to shred the flesh into strands.

Empty the spaghetti strands into a bowl and mix with butter, garlic powder,

chili powder, coconut cream, cream cheese, half of mozzarella cheese, and

Parmesan cheese. Spoon the mixture into the squash cups and sprinkle with

the remaining mozzarella cheese. Bake further for 5 minutes or until the

cheese is golden brown. Sprinkle with cilantro and serve.

Per serving: Cal 515; Net Carbs 7g; Fat 45g; Protein 18g

Asparagus with Creamy Puree

Ingredients for 4 servings

4 tbsp flax seed powder

5 oz butter, melted

3 oz grated cashew cheese

½ cup coconut cream

1 tbsp olive oil

½ lb asparagus, stalks removed

Juice of ½ lemon

½ tsp chili pepper

Instructions - Total Time: around 15 minutes

In a bowl, mix flax seed powder with ½ cup water and set aside for 5

minutes. Warm the flax egg in the microwave for 2 minutes, then, pour into a

blender. Add in 2 oz butter, coconut cream, salt, and chili pepper; puree until

smooth.

Place a grill pan over medium heat. Brush the asparagus with olive oil and

cook in the pan until lightly charred. Set aside. Warm the remaining butter in

a frying pan until nutty and golden brown. Stir in lemon juice and pour the

mixture into a sauce cup. Spoon the creamy blend into four plates and spread

out lightly. Top with asparagus and drizzle the lemon butter on top. Serve.

Per serving: Cal 520g; Net Carbs 6g; Fat 53g; Protein 6.3g

Grilled Zucchini with Spinach Avocado Pesto

Ingredients for 4 servings

3 oz spinach, chopped

1 avocado, chopped

Juice of 1 lemon

1 garlic clove, minced

2 oz pecans

Salt and black pepper to taste

¾ cup olive oil

2 zucchinis, sliced

2 tbsp melted butter

Instructions - Total Time: around 20 minutes

Place spinach in a food processor along with avocado, half of lemon juice,

garlic, olive oil, and pecans and blend until smooth; season with salt and pepper. Pour the pesto into a bowl and set aside. Season zucchini with the

remaining lemon juice, salt, pepper, and butter. Preheat a grill pan and cook

the zucchini slices until browned. Remove to a plate, spoon the pesto to the

side, and serve.

Per serving: Cal 550; Net Carbs 6g; Fat 46g; Protein 25g

Greek-Style Pizza

Ingredients for 4 servings

½ cup almond flour

¼ tsp salt

2 tbsp ground psyllium husk

1 tbsp olive oil

¼ tsp red chili flakes

¼ tsp dried Greek seasoning

1 cup crumbled feta cheese

3 plum tomatoes, sliced

6 Kalamata olives, chopped

5 basil leaves, chopped

Instructions - Total Time: around 30 minutes

Preheat oven to 390 F. Line a baking sheet with parchment paper. In a bowl,

mix almond flour, salt, psyllium powder, olive oil, and 1 cup of lukewarm water until dough forms.

Spread the mixture on the baking sheet and bake for 10 minutes. Sprinkle the

red chili flakes and Greek seasoning on the crust and top with the feta cheese.

Arrange the tomatoes and olives on top. Bake for 10 minutes. Garnish the

pizza with basil, slice, and serve warm.

Per serving: Cal 276; Net Carbs 4.5g; Fats 12g; Protein 8g

Sweet & Spicy Brussels Sprout Stir-Fry

Ingredients for 4 servings

2 tbsp butter

2 shallots, chopped

1 tbsp apple cider vinegar

Salt and black pepper to taste

2 cups Brussels sprouts, halved

1 tbsp hot chili sauce

Instructions - Total Time: around 15 minutes

Melt the butter in a saucepan over medium heat and sauté shallots for 2

minutes until slightly soften. Add in apple cider vinegar, salt, and pepper. Stir

and reduce the heat. Continue cooking the shallots with continuous stirring,

about 5 minutes. Transfer to a plate.

Pour Brussels sprouts into the saucepan and stir-fry

for 5 minutes. Season

with salt and pepper, stir in shallots and hot chili sauce, and heat for a few

seconds. Serve.

Per serving: Cal 260; Net Carbs 7g; Fat 23g; Protein 3g

Eggplant Fries with Chili Aioli & Beet Salad

Ingredients for 4 servings

1 egg, beaten in a bowl

2 eggplants, sliced

2 cups almond flour

Salt and black pepper to taste

2 tbsp butter, melted

2 egg yolks

2 garlic cloves, minced

1 cup olive oil

½ tsp red chili flakes

2 tbsp lemon juice

3 tbsp yogurt

3 ½ oz cooked beets, shredded

3 ½ oz red cabbage, shredded

2 tbsp fresh cilantro, chopped

Instructions - Total Time: around 25 minutes

Preheat oven to 400 F. In a deep plate, mix flour, salt, and pepper. Dip

eggplants into the egg, then in the flour. Place on a greased baking sheet and

brush with butter. Bake for 15 minutes. To make aioli whisk egg yolks with

garlic. Gradually pour in ¾ cup olive oil while whisking. Stir in chili flakes,

salt, pepper, 1 tbsp of lemon juice, and yogurt. In a salad bowl, mix beets,

cabbage, cilantro, remaining oil, remaining lemon juice, salt, and pepper; toss

to coat. Serve the fries with the chili aioli and beet salad.

Per serving: Cal 850; Net Carbs 8g; Fat 77g; Protein 26g

Creamy Brussels Sprout Bake

Ingredients for 4 servings

3 tbsp butter

1 lb chicken breasts, cubed

1½ lb halved Brussels sprouts

5 garlic cloves, minced

1¼ cups coconut cream

2 cups grated cheddar

¼ cup grated Parmesan

Salt and black pepper to taste

Instructions - Total Time: around 40 minutes

Preheat oven to 400 F. Melt butter in a skillet and sauté chicken cubes for 6

minutes; remove to a plate. Pour the Brussels sprouts and garlic into the

skillet and sauté until nice color forms. Mix in coconut cream and simmer for

4 minutes. Mix in chicken cubes. Pour the sauté into

a baking dish, sprinkle

with cheddar and Parmesan cheeses. Bake for 10 minutes. Serve with tomato

salad.

Per serving: Cal 420; Net Carbs 7g; Fat 34g; Protein 13g

Mushroom Lettuce Wraps

Ingredients for 4 servings

4 oz baby bella mushrooms, sliced

1 iceberg lettuce, leaves extracted

1 cup grated cheddar cheese

2 tbsp butter

1 lb goat cheese, crumbled

Salt and black pepper to taste

1 large tomato, sliced

Instructions - Total Time: around 20 minutes

Melt butter in a skillet over medium heat. Add mushrooms and sauté until

tender, 6 minutes. Add in goat cheese and cook for 5 minutes, stirring

occasionally. Spoon the mixture into the lettuce leaves, sprinkle with cheddar

cheese, and top with tomato slices. Serve immediately.

Per serving: Cal 620; Net Carbs 3g; Fat 52g; Protein 32g

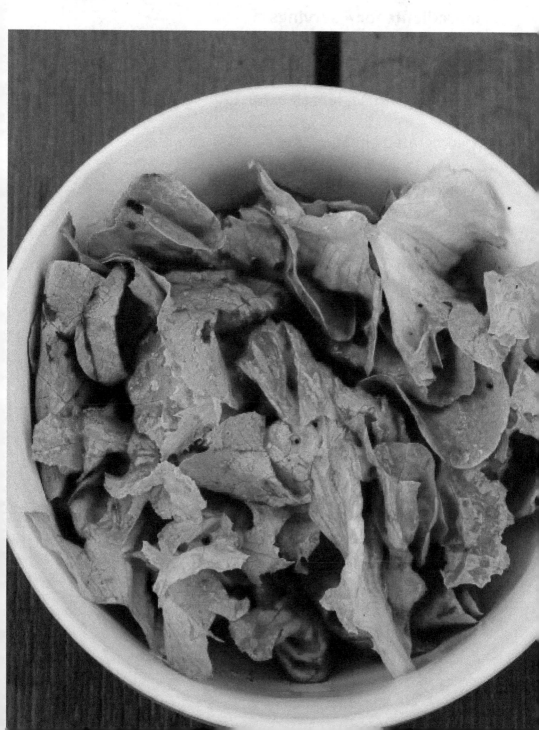

Cheesy Cauliflower Casserole

Ingredients for 4 servings

2 oz butter, melted

1 white onion, finely chopped

½ cup celery stalks, chopped

1 green bell pepper, chopped

1 head cauliflower, chopped

1 cup mayonnaise

4 oz grated Parmesan

1 tsp red chili flakes

Instructions - Total Time: around 35 minutes

Preheat oven to 400 F. In a bowl, mix cauliflower, mayonnaise, butter, and

chili flakes. Pour the mixture into a greased baking dish and distribute the

onion, celery, and bell pepper evenly on top. Sprinkle with Parmesan cheese

and bake until golden, 20 minutes. Serve.

Per serving: Cal 464; Net Carbs 4g; Fat 37g; Protein 36g

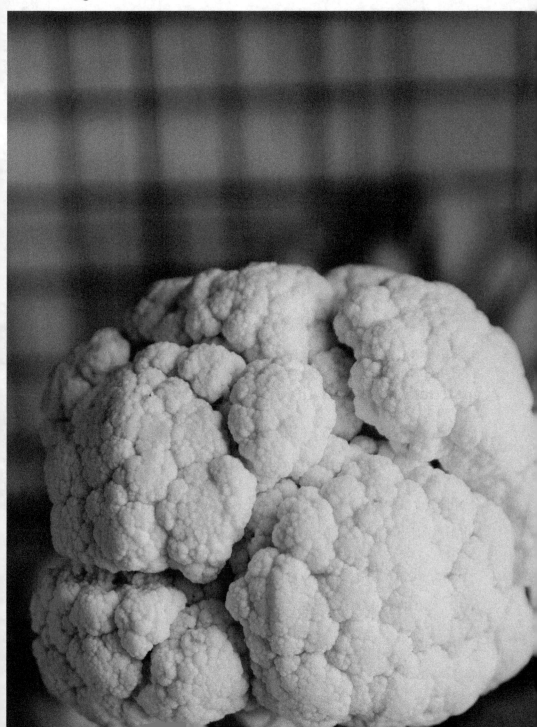

Baked Stuffed Avocados

Ingredients for 4 servings

3 avocados, halved and pitted, skin on

½ cup mozzarella, shredded

½ cup Swiss cheese, grated

2 eggs, beaten

1 tbsp fresh cilantro, chopped

Instructions - Total Time: around 20 minutes

Set oven to 360 F. Lay avocado halves in an ovenproof dish. In a bowl, mix

both types of cheeses and eggs. Split the mixture into the avocado halves.

Bake for 15 to 17 minutes. Decorate with cilantro before serving.

Per serving: Cal 342; Net Carbs: 7g; Fat: 30g; Protein: 11g

Garam Masala Pork Bake

Ingredients for 4 servings

3 tbsp butter

1 lb ground pork

2 tbsp garam masala

1 green bell pepper, diced

1 ¼ cups coconut cream

1 tbsp fresh cilantro, chopped

Instructions - Total Time: around 30 minutes

Preheat oven to 400 F. Melt butter in a skillet and brown the ground pork for

about 4 minutes. Stir in garam masala. Transfer the mixture to a baking dish.

Mix in bell pepper, coconut cream, and cilantro and bake for 20 minutes.

Per serving: Cal 610; Net Carbs 5g; Fat 47g; Protein 35g

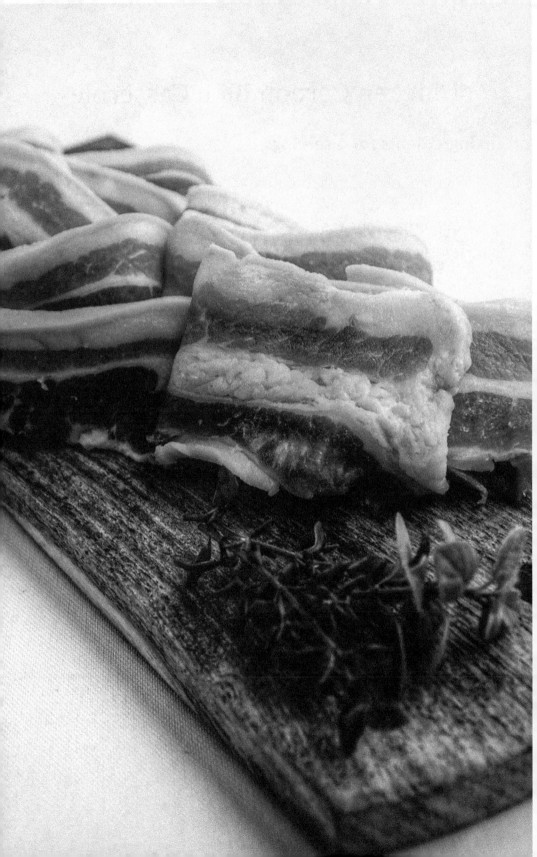

Chicken Cordon Bleu Casserole

Ingredients for 4 servings

1 lb chicken breasts, cubed

1 cup cream cheese

1 tbsp mustard powder

1 tbsp plain vinegar

1 ¼ cups grated cheddar

½ cup baby spinach

Instructions - Total Time: around 30 minutes

Preheat oven to 400 F. Mix cream cheese, mustard powder, plain vinegar,

chicken, and cheddar cheese in a greased baking dish. Bake until golden

brown, about 20 minutes. Serve warm.

Per serving: Cal 980; Net Carbs 6g; Fat 92g; Protein 30g

Zoodle Bolognese

Ingredients for 4 servings

3 oz olive oil

1 white onion, chopped

1 garlic clove, minced

1 carrot, chopped

½ lb ground pork

2 tbsp tomato paste

1 ½ cups crushed tomatoes

Salt and black pepper to taste

1 tbsp dried basil

1 tbsp Worcestershire sauce

2 lbs zucchini, spiralized

2 tbsp butter

Instructions - Total Time: around 45 minutes

Heat olive oil in a saucepan and sauté onion, garlic, and carrot for 3 minutes.

Pour in ground pork, tomato paste, tomatoes, salt, pepper, basil, some water,

and Worcestershire sauce. Stir and cook for 15 minutes. Melt butter in a

skillet and toss in zoodles quickly, about 1 minute; season. Serve the zoodles

topped with the sauce.

Per serving: Cal 425; Net Carbs 6g; Fat 33g; Protein 20g

Baked Tofu with Roasted Peppers

Ingredients for 4 servings

3 oz cream cheese

¾ cup mayonnaise

1 cucumber, diced

1 large tomato, chopped

Salt and black pepper to taste

1 tsp dried parsley

4 orange bell peppers

2 ½ cups cubed tofu

1 tbsp melted butter

1 tsp dried basil

Instructions - Total Time: around 20 minutes

Preheat a broiler to 450 F. Line a baking sheet with parchment paper. In a

salad bowl, combine cream cheese, mayonnaise, cucumber, tomato, salt, pepper, and parsley; refrigerate. Arrange bell peppers and tofu on the paperlined

baking sheet, drizzle with melted butter, and season with basil, salt, and

pepper. Use hands to rub the ingredients until evenly coated. Bake for 15

minutes until the peppers have charred lightly and the tofu browned.

Per serving: Cal 840; Net Carbs 8g; Fat 76g; Protein 28g

Spicy Cheese Balls

Ingredients for 4 servings

1/3 cup mayonnaise

¼ cup pickled jalapenos

1 tsp paprika

1 tbsp mustard powder

1 pinch of cayenne pepper

4 oz grated cheddar

1 tbsp flax seed powder

2 ½ cups crumbled feta

Salt and black pepper to taste

2 tbsp butter

Instructions - Total Time: around 40 minutes

In a bowl, mix mayonnaise, jalapenos, paprika, mustard, cayenne, and

cheddar cheese; set aside. In another bowl, combine flax seed powder with 3 tbsp water and allow absorbing for 5 minutes. Add the flax egg to the cheese

mixture, crumbled feta, salt, and pepper; mix well. Form balls out of the mix.

Melt butter in a skillet over medium heat and fry balls until cooked and

browned on the outside.

Per serving: Cal 650; Net Carbs 2g; Fat 52g; Protein 43g

Zucchini Boats with Cheddar Cheese

Ingredients for 2 servings

1 zucchini, halved

4 tbsp butter

2 garlic cloves, minced

1½ oz baby kale

Salt and black pepper to taste

2 tbsp tomato sauce

1 cup cheddar cheese

Instructions - Total Time: around 40 minutes

Preheat oven to 375 F. Scoop out zucchini pulp with a spoon. Keep the flesh.

Grease a baking sheet with cooking spray and place in the zucchini boats.

Melt butter in a skillet over medium heat and sauté garlic until fragrant and

slightly browned, 4 minutes.

Add in kale and zucchini pulp. Cook until the kale wilts; season with salt and

pepper. Spoon tomato sauce into the boats and spread to coat evenly. Spoon

kale mixture into the zucchinis and sprinkle with cheddar cheese. Bake for 25

minutes.

Per serving: Cal 620; Net Carbs 4g; Fat 57g; Protein 20g

Roasted Butternut Squash with Chimichurri

Ingredients for 4 servings

Zest and juice of 1 lemon

½ red bell pepper, chopped

1 jalapeño pepper, chopped

1 cup olive oil

½ cup chopped fresh parsley

2 garlic cloves, minced

Salt and black pepper to taste

1 lb butternut squash

1 tbsp butter, melted

3 tbsp toasted pine nuts

Instructions - Total Time: around 15 minutes

In a bowl, add lemon zest and juice, bell pepper, jalapeño, olive oil, parsley,

garlic, salt, and pepper. Use an immersion blender to

grind the ingredients

until desired consistency is achieved; set chimichurri aside. Slice the squash

into rounds and remove the seeds. Drizzle with butter and season with salt

and pepper. Preheat grill pan over medium heat and cook the squash for 2

minutes on each side. Scatter pine nuts on top and serve with chimichurri.

Per serving: Cal 650; Net Carbs 6g; Fat 44g; Protein 55g

Roasted Chorizo with Mixed Greens

Ingredients for 4 servings

1 lb chorizo, sliced

1 lb asparagus, halved

2 mixed bell peppers, diced

1 cup green beans, trimmed

2 red onions, cut into wedges

1 head broccoli, cut into florets

Salt and black pepper to taste

4 tbsp olive oil

1 tbsp sugar-free maple syrup

1 lemon, juiced

Instructions - Total Time: around 30 minutes

Preheat oven to 400 F. On a baking tray, add chorizo, asparagus, bell

peppers, green beans, onions, and broccoli and

season with salt, pepper.

Drizzle with oil and maple syrup. Bake for 15 minutes. Top with lemon juice.

Per serving: Cal 300; Net Carbs 3.3g; Fat 18g; Protein 15g

Baked Eggplants with Tomato Sauce

Ingredients for 4 servings

2 eggplants, sliced

1/3 cup melted butter

2 garlic cloves, minced

1 red onion, sliced

7 oz tomato sauce

2 tbsp Parmesan, grated

Salt and black pepper to taste

¼ cup chopped fresh parsley

Instructions - Total Time: around 25 minutes

Preheat oven to 400 F. Line a baking sheet with parchment paper. Brush

eggplants with butter. Bake until lightly browned, 20 minutes.

Heat the remaining butter in a skillet and sauté garlic and onion until fragrant and soft, about 3 minutes. Stir in tomato sauce and season with salt and

pepper. Simmer for 10 minutes. Remove eggplants from the oven and spread

the tomato sauce on top. Sprinkle with Parmesan cheese and parsley and

serve.

Per serving: Cal 600; Net Carbs 12g; Fat 46g; Protein 26g

Tomato Artichoke Pizza

Ingredients for 4 servings

2 oz canned artichokes, cut into wedges

2 eggs

1 cup grated broccoli

1 cup grated Parmesan

½ tsp salt

2 tbsp tomato sauce

½ cup mozzarella, grated

1 garlic clove, thinly sliced

½ tbsp dried oregano

Green olives for garnish

Instructions - Total Time: around 40 minutes

Preheat oven to 350 F. Line a baking sheet with parchment paper. In a bowl,

add broccoli, eggs, and Parmesan cheese, and stir to combine. Pour the mixture into the baking sheet and bake until the crust is lightly browned, 20

minutes. Remove from oven and spread tomato sauce on top, sprinkle with

mozzarella cheese, add artichokes and garlic. Spread oregano on top. Bake

pizza for 10 minutes. Garnish with olives and serve.

Per serving: Cal 860; Net Carbs 10g; Fat 63g; Protein 55g

Seitan Cauliflower Gratin

Ingredients for 4 servings

2 oz butter

1 leek, coarsely chopped

1 onion, coarsely chopped

2 cups broccoli florets

1 cup cauliflower florets

2 cups crumbled seitan

1 cup coconut cream

2 tbsp mustard powder

5 oz grated Parmesan

4 tbsp fresh rosemary

Instructions - Total Time: around 40 minutes

Preheat oven to 450 F. Put half of butter in a pot over medium heat to melt.

Add leek, onion, broccoli, and cauliflower and cook until the vegetables have softened, about 6 minutes. Transfer them to a baking dish. Melt the remaining

butter in a skillet over medium heat, and cook seitan until browned.

Mix coconut cream and mustard powder in a bowl. Pour mixture over the

veggies. Scatter seitan and Parmesan on top and sprinkle with rosemary.

Bake for 15 minutes.

Per serving: Cal 480; Net Carbs 9.8g; Fat 40g; Protein 16g

Curry Cauli Rice with Mushrooms

Ingredients for 4 servings

8 oz baby bella mushrooms, stemmed and sliced

2 heads cauliflower, chopped

2 tbsp sesame oil

1 onion, chopped

3 garlic cloves, minced

Salt and black pepper to taste

½ tsp curry powder

1 tsp chopped parsley

2 scallions, thinly sliced

Instructions - Total Time: around 15 minutes

Place cauliflower in a food processor and pulse until rice-like consistency.

Heat sesame oil in a skillet over medium heat and sauté onion, garlic, and mushrooms for 5 minutes until the mushrooms are soft.

Pour in cauli rice and cook for 6 minutes. Season with salt, pepper, and curry

powder. Remove from heat. Stir in parsley and scallions and serve.

Per serving: Cal 305; Net Carbs 7g; Fat 25g; Protein 6g

Parmesan Meatballs

Ingredients for 4 servings

½ lb ground beef

½ lb ground Italian sausage

¾ cup pork rinds

½ cup grated Parmesan cheese

2 eggs

1 tsp onion powder

1 tsp garlic powder

1 tbsp chopped fresh basil

Salt and black pepper to taste

2 tsp dried Italian seasoning

3 tbsp olive oil

2 ½ cups marinara sauce

Instructions - Total Time: around 1 hour

In a bowl, add beef, Italian sausage, pork rinds, Parmesan cheese, eggs, onion powder, garlic powder, basil, salt, pepper, and Italian seasoning. Form

meatballs out of the mixture. Heat the remaining olive oil in a skillet and

brown the meatballs for 10 minutes. Pour in marinara sauce and submerge the

meatballs in the sauce; cook for 45 minutes.

Per serving: Cal 513; Net Carbs 8.2g; Fat 24g; Protein 35g

White Pizza with Mixed Mushrooms

Ingredients for 4 servings

2 tbsp flax seed powder

½ cup mayonnaise

¾ cup almond flour

1 tbsp psyllium husk powder

1 tsp baking powder

2 oz mixed mushrooms, sliced

1 tbsp basil pesto

½ cup coconut cream

¾ cup grated Parmesan

Instructions - Total Time: around 35 minutes

Preheat oven to 350 F. Combine flax seed powder with 6 tbsp water and

allow sitting for 5 minutes. Whisk in mayonnaise, almond flour, psyllium husk, and baking powder; let rest. Pour batter into a baking sheet.

Bake for 10 minutes. In a bowl, mix mushrooms with pesto. Remove crust

from the oven and spread coconut cream on top. Add the mushroom mixture

and Parmesan cheese. Bake the pizza further until the cheese melts, about 5-

10 minutes. Slice and serve.

Per serving: Cal 750; Net Carbs 6g; Fat 69g; Protein 22g

Arugula & Pecan Pizza

Ingredients for 4 servings

½ cup almond flour

2 tbsp ground psyllium husk

1 tbsp olive oil

1 cup basil pesto

1 cup grated mozzarella

1 tomato, thinly sliced

1 zucchini, cut into half-moons

1 cup baby arugula

2 tbsp chopped pecans

¼ tsp red chili flakes

Instructions - Total Time: around 30 minutes

Preheat oven to 390 F. Line a baking sheet with parchment paper. In a bowl,

mix almond flour, psyllium powder, olive oil, and 1 cup of lukewarm water until dough forms. Spread the mixture on the sheet and bake for 10 minutes.

Spread pesto on the crust and top with mozzarella cheese, tomato slices, and

zucchini. Bake until the cheese melts, 15 minutes. Top with arugula, pecans,

and red chili flakes.

Per serving: Cal 186; Net Carbs 3g; Fats 14g; Protein 11g

Pepperoni Fat Head Pizza

Ingredients for 4 servings

1 ½ cups grated mozzarella

2 tbsp cream cheese, softened

1 eggs, beaten

¾ cup almond flour

1 tsp dried oregano

4 tbsp tomato sauce

½ cup sliced pepperoni

Instructions - Total Time: around 35 minutes

Preheat oven to 420 F. Line a round pizza pan with parchment paper.

Microwave the mozzarella cheese and cream cheese for 1 minute. Stir in egg

and add in the almond flour; mix well. Transfer the pizza "dough" onto a flat

surface and knead until smooth. Spread it on the pizza pan. Bake for 6 minutes. Top with tomato sauce, remaining mozzarella, oregano, and

pepperoni. Bake for 15 minutes. Serve sliced.

Per serving: Cal 229; Net Carbs 0.4g; Fats 7g; Protein 36g

Walnut Stuffed Mushrooms

Ingredients for 4 servings

½ cup grated Pecorino Romano cheese

12 button mushrooms, stemmed

¼ cup pork rinds

2 garlic cloves, minced

2 tbsp chopped fresh parsley

Salt and black pepper to taste

¼ cup ground walnuts

¼ cup olive oil

Instructions - Total Time: around 30 minutes

Preheat oven to 400 F. In a bowl, mix pork rinds, Pecorino Romano cheese,

garlic, parsley, salt, and pepper.

Brush a baking sheet with some oil. Spoon the cheese mixture into the

mushrooms and arrange on the baking sheet. Top with the ground walnuts and drizzle the remaining olive oil on the mushrooms. Bake for 20 minutes or

until golden. Transfer to a platter and serve.

Per serving: Cal 292; Net Carbs 7.1g; Fat 25g; Protein 8g

Cheese & Beef Avocado Boats

Ingredients for 4 servings

2 tbsp avocado oil

1 lb ground beef

Salt and black pepper to taste

1 tsp onion powder

1 tsp cumin powder

1 tsp garlic powder

2 tsp taco seasoning

2 tsp smoked paprika

1 cup raw pecans, chopped

1 tbsp hemp seeds, hulled

7 tbsp shredded Monterey Jack

2 avocados, halved and pitted

1 medium tomato, sliced

¼ cup shredded iceberg lettuce

4 tbsp sour cream

4 tbsp shredded Monterey Jack

Instructions - Total Time: around 30 minutes

Heat half of avocado oil in a skillet and cook beef for 10 minutes. Season

with salt, pepper, onion powder, cumin, garlic, taco seasoning, and smoked

paprika. Add the pecans and hemp seeds and stir-fry for 10 minutes. Fold in 3

tbsp Monterey Jack cheese to melt. Spoon the filling into avocado holes, top

with 1-2 slices of tomatoes, some lettuce, 1 tbsp each of sour cream, and the

remaining Monterey Jack cheese and serve immediately.

Per serving: Cal 840; Net Carbs 4g; Fat 70g; Protein 42g

Celery & Beef Stuffed Mushrooms

Ingredients for 4 servings

½ cup shredded Pecorino Romano cheese

2 tbsp olive oil

½ celery stalk, chopped

1 shallot, finely chopped

1 lb ground beef

2 tbsp mayonnaise

1 tsp Old Bay seasoning

½ tsp garlic powder

2 large eggs

4 caps Portobello mushrooms

1 tbsp flaxseed meal

2 tbsp shredded Parmesan

1 tbsp chopped parsley

Instructions - Total Time: around 55 minutes

Preheat oven to 350 F. Heat olive oil in a skillet and

sauté celery and shallot

for 3 minutes; set aside. Add beef to the skillet and cook for 10 minutes; add

to the shallot mixture. Pour in mayonnaise, Old Bay seasoning, garlic

powder, Pecorino cheese and crack in the eggs. Combine the mixture evenly.

Arrange the mushrooms on a greased baking sheet and fill with the meat

mixture. Combine flaxseed meal and Parmesan cheese in a bowl and sprinkle

over the mushroom filling. Bake until the cheese melts, 30 minutes. Garnish

with parsley to serve.

Per serving: Cal 375; Net Carbs 3.5g; Fat 22g; Protein 37g

Herby Beef Meatza

Ingredients for 4 servings

1 ½ lb ground beef

Salt and black pepper to taste

1 large egg

1 tsp rosemary

1 tsp thyme

3 garlic cloves, minced

1 tsp basil

½ tbsp oregano

¾ cup low-carb tomato sauce

¼ cup shredded Parmesan

1 cup shredded Pepper Jack

1 cup shredded mozzarella

Instructions - Total Time: around 30 minutes

Preheat oven to 350 F. In a bowl, combine beef, salt, pepper, egg, rosemary, thyme, garlic, basil, and oregano. Transfer the mixture into a greased baking

pan and using hands, flatten to a two-inch thickness. Bake for 15 minutes

until the beef has a lightly brown crust. Remove and spread tomato sauce on

top. Sprinkle with Parmesan, Pepper Jack, and mozzarella cheeses. Return to

oven to bake until the cheeses melt, 5 minutes. Serve.

Per serving: Cal 319; Net Carbs 3.6g; Fat 10g; Protein 49g

Homemade Pasta with Meatballs

Ingredients for 4 servings

1 cup shredded mozzarella

1 egg yolk

½ cup olive oil

1 yellow onion, chopped

6 garlic cloves, minced

2 tbsp tomato paste

2 large tomatoes, chopped

¼ tsp saffron powder

2 cinnamon sticks

1 cup chicken broth

Salt and black pepper to taste

1 cup pork rinds

1 lb ground beef

1 egg

¼ cup almond milk

¼ tsp nutmeg powder

1 tbsp smoked paprika

1 ½ tsp fresh ginger paste

1 tsp cumin powder

½ tsp cayenne pepper

½ tsp clove powder

4 tbsp chopped cilantro

4 tbsp chopped scallions

4 tbsp chopped parsley

¼ cup almond flour

1 cup crumbled feta cheese

Instructions - Total Time: around 40 min + chilling time

Microwave mozzarella cheese for 2 minutes. Mix in egg yolk until combined.

Lay parchment paper on a flat surface, pour the cheese mixture on top and

cover with another piece of parchment paper. Flatten

the dough into 1/8-inch

thickness. Take off the parchment paper.

Cut the dough into spaghetti strands; refrigerate overnight. When ready, bring

2 cups of water to a boil in a saucepan and add the " pasta". Cook for 1

minute, drain, and let cool. In a pot, heat 2 tbsp of olive oil and sauté onion

and half of the garlic for 3 minutes. Stir in tomato paste, tomatoes, saffron,

and cinnamon sticks; cook for 2 minutes. Mix in chicken broth, salt, and

pepper. Simmer for 10 minutes.

In a bowl, mix pork rinds, beef, egg, almond milk, remaining garlic, salt,

pepper, nutmeg, paprika, ginger, cumin, cayenne, clove powder, cilantro,

parsley, 3 tbsp of scallions, and almond flour. Form balls out of the mixture.

Heat the remaining olive oil in a skillet and fry the meatballs for 10 minutes.

Place them into the sauce and continue cooking for 5-10 minutes. Divide the

pasta onto serving plates and spoon the meatballs with sauce on top. Garnish

with feta cheese and scallions and serve.

Per serving: Cal 783; Net Carbs 6g; Fats 56g; Protein 55g

Morning Beef Bowl

Ingredients for 4 servings

1 lb beef sirloin, cut into strips

¼ cup tamari sauce

2 tbsp lemon juice

3 tsp garlic powder

1 tbsp swerve sugar

2 tbsp coconut oil

6 garlic cloves, minced

1 lb cauliflower rice

2 tbsp olive oil

4 large eggs

2 tbsp chopped scallions

Instructions - Total Time: around 35 min + chilling time

In a bowl, mix tamari sauce, lemon juice, garlic powder, and swerve sugar.

Pour beef into a zipper bag and add in the mixture. Massage the meat to coat

well. Refrigerate overnight. The next day, heat coconut oil in a wok, and fry

the beef until the liquid evaporates and the meat cooks through, 12 minutes;

set aside. Sauté garlic for 1 minute in the same wok. Mix in cauli rice until

softened, 5 minutes. Spoon into 4 serving bowls and set aside. Wipe the wok

clean and heat 1 tbsp of olive oil. Crack in two eggs and fry sunshine-style, 1

minute. Place an egg on each cauliflower rice bowl and fry the other 2 eggs

with the remaining olive oil. Serve garnished with scallions.

Per serving: Cal 908; Net Carbs 5.1g; Fat 83g; Protein 34g

Homemade Philly Cheesesteak in Omelet

Ingredients for 2 servings

4 large eggs

2 tbsp almond milk

2 tbsp olive oil

1 yellow onion, sliced

½ green bell pepper, sliced

¼ lb beef ribeye shaved steak

Salt and black pepper to taste

2 oz provolone cheese, sliced

Instructions - Total Time: around 35 minutes

In a bowl, beat the eggs with milk. Heat half of the oil in a skillet and pour in

half of the eggs. Fry until cooked on one side, flip, and cook until well done.

Slide into a plate and fry the remaining eggs. Place them into another plate.

Heat the remaining olive oil in the same skillet and sauté the onion and bell

pepper for 5 minutes; set aside. Season beef with salt and pepper and cook it

in the skillet until brown with no crust. Add onion and pepper back to the

skillet and cook for 1 minute. Lay provolone cheese in the omelet and top

with the hot meat mixture. Roll the eggs and place back to the skillet to melt

the cheese. Serve.

Per serving: Cal 497; Net Carbs 3.6g; Fat 36g; Protein 34g

Korean Braised Beef with Kelp Noodles

Ingredients for 4 servings

1 ½ lb sirloin steak, cut into strips

2 (16- oz) packs kelp noodles, thoroughly rinsed

1 tbsp coconut oil

2 pieces star anise

1 cinnamon stick

1 garlic clove, minced

1-inch ginger, grated

3 tbsp coconut aminos

2 tbsp swerve brown sugar

¼ cup red wine

4 cups beef broth

1 head napa cabbage, steamed

2 tbsp scallions, thinly sliced

Instructions - Total Time: around 2 hours 15

minutes

Heat oil in a pot over and sauté anise, cinnamon, garlic, and ginger until

fragrant, 5 minutes. Add in beef and sear it on both sides, 10 minutes. In a

bowl, combine aminos, swerve brown sugar, red wine, and ¼ cup water. Pour

the mixture into the pot, close the lid, and bring to a boil. Reduce the heat and

simmer for 1 to 1 ½ hours or until the meat is tender. Strain the pot's content

through a colander into a bowl and pour the braising liquid back into the pot.

Discard cinnamon and anise and set aside. Add beef broth and simmer for 10

minutes. Put kelp noodles in the broth and cook until softened and separated,

6 minutes. Spoon the noodles and some broth into bowls, add beef strips, and

top with cabbage and scallions.

Per serving: Cal 548; Net Carbs 26g; Fat 27g; Protein 44g

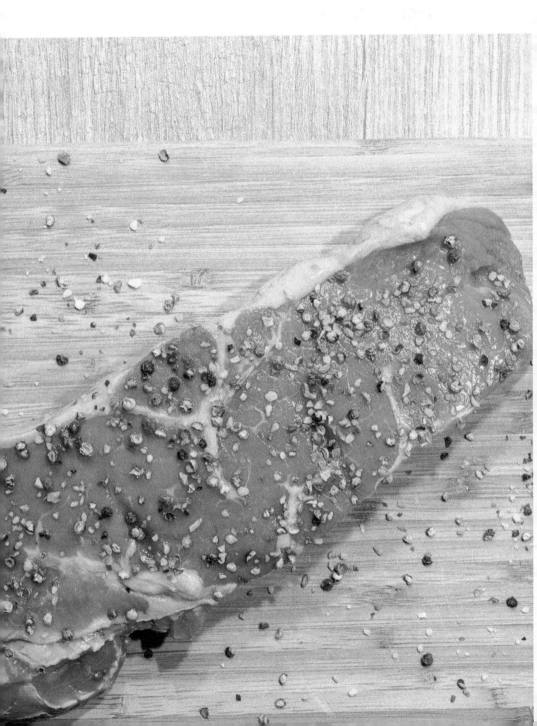

Habanero Beef Cauliflower Pilaf

Ingredients for 4 servings

2 tbsp olive oil

½ lb ground beef

Salt and black pepper to taste

1 yellow onion, chopped

2 garlic cloves, minced

1 habanero pepper, minced

½ tsp Italian seasoning

2 ½ cups cauliflower rice

2 tbsp tomato paste

½ cup beef broth

¼ cup chopped parsley

1 lemon, sliced

Instructions - Total Time: around 30 minutes

Warm olive oil in a skillet over medium heat and cook
the beef until no

longer brown, 8 minutes. Season with salt and pepper and spoon into a plate.

In the same skillet, sauté onion, garlic, and habanero pepper for 2 minutes.

Mix in Italian seasoning, cauli rice, tomato paste, and broth. Season to taste

and cook for 10 minutes. Mix in beef for 3 minutes. Garnish with parsley and

lemon. Serve.

Per serving: Cal 216; Net Carbs 3.8g; Fat 14g; Protein 15g

Balsamic Meatloaf

Ingredients for 4 servings

1 pounds ground beef

1 onion, chopped

¼ cup almond flour

2 garlic cloves, minced

¼ cup mushrooms, sliced

1 egg

2 tbsp parsley, chopped

¼ cup chopped bell peppers

2 tbsp grated Parmesan

½ tsp balsamic vinegar

Glaze:

1 cup balsamic vinegar

1 tbsp sweetener

1 tbsp sugar-free ketchup

Instructions - Total Time: around 1 hour 15

minutes

Combine all meatloaf ingredients in a large bowl. Press the mixture into a

greased loaf pan. Bake in preheated oven at 370 F for about 30 minutes.

Combine all glaze ingredients in a saucepan over medium heat. Simmer for

10 minutes or until the glaze thickens. Spread some glaze over the meatloaf.

Save the extra for future use. Put the meatloaf back in the oven and cook for

5 minutes. Serve.

Per serving: Cal 264; Net Carbs 6g; Fat 19g; Protein 23g

Mustard Beef Collard Rolls

Ingredients for 4 servings

2 lb corned beef

1 tbsp butter

Salt and black pepper to taste

2 tsp Worcestershire sauce

1 tsp Dijon mustard

1 tsp whole peppercorns

¼ tsp cloves

¼ tsp allspice

½ tsp red pepper flakes

1 large bay leaf

1 lemon, zested and juiced

¼ cup white wine

¼ cup freshly brewed coffee

2/3 tbsp swerve sugar

8 large Swiss collard leaves

1 medium red onion, sliced

Instructions - Total Time: around 70 minutes

In a pot, add beef, butter, salt, pepper, Worcestershire sauce, mustard,

peppercorns, cloves, allspice, red pepper flakes, bay leaf, lemon zest, lemon

juice, white wine, coffee, and swerve sugar. Close the lid and cook over low

heat for 1 hour. Ten minutes before the end, bring a pot of water to a boil,

add collards with one slice of onion for 30 seconds and transfer to ice bath;

let sit for 2-3 minutes. Remove, pat dry, and lay on a flat surface. Remove the

meat from the pot, place on a cutting board, and slice. Divide meat between

the collards, top with onion slices, and roll the leaves. Serve with tomato

gravy.

Per serving: Cal 349; Net Carbs 1.5g; Fat 16g; Protein 47g

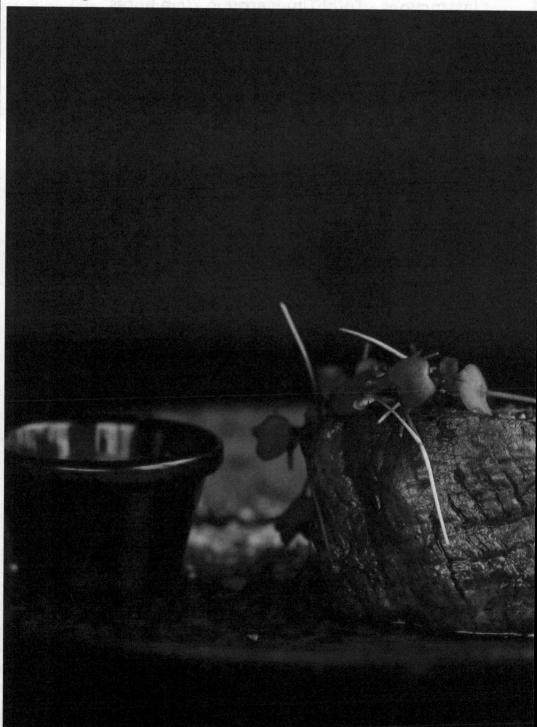

Beef Alfredo Squash Spaghetti

Ingredients for 4 servings

2 medium spaghetti squashes, halved

2 tbsp olive oil

2 tbsp butter

1 lb ground beef

½ tsp garlic powder

Salt and black pepper to taste

1 tsp arrowroot starch

1 ½ cups heavy cream

A pinch of nutmeg

1/3 cup grated Parmesan

1/3 cup grated mozzarella

Instructions - Total Time: around 1 hour 20 minutes

Preheat oven to 375 F. Drizzle the squash with olive oil and season with salt and pepper. Place on a lined with foil baking dish and roast for 45 minutes.

Let cool and shred the inner part of the noodles; set aside.

Melt butter in a pot over medium heat, add in beef, garlic powder, salt, and

pepper, and cook for 10 minutes, stirring often. Stir in arrowroot starch,

heavy cream, and nutmeg. Cook until the sauce thickens, 2-3 minutes. Spoon

the sauce into the squashes and cover with Parmesan and mozzarella cheeses.

Cook under the broiler for 3 minutes.

Per serving: Cal 563; Net Carbs 4g; Fats 42g; Protein 36g

Kentucky Cauliflower with Mashed Parsnips

Ingredients for 6 servings

½ cup almond milk

¼ cup coconut flour

¼ tsp cayenne pepper

½ cup almond breadcrumbs

½ cup grated cheddar cheese

30 oz cauliflower florets

1 lb parsnips, quartered

3 tbsp melted butter

A pinch nutmeg

1 tsp cumin powder

1 cup coconut cream

2 tbsp sesame oil

Instructions - Total Time: around 35 minutes

Preheat oven to 425 F. Line a baking sheet with

parchment paper. In a bowl,

combine almond milk, coconut flour, and cayenne. In another bowl, mix

breadcrumbs and cheddar cheese. Dip each cauliflower floret into the milk

mixture, and then into the cheese mixture.

Place breaded cauliflower on the baking sheet and bake for 30 minutes,

turning once. Pour 4 cups of slightly salted water in a pot and add in parsnips.

Bring to boil and cook for 15 minutes. Drain and transfer to a bowl.

Add in melted butter, cumin, nutmeg, and coconut cream. Mash the

ingredients using a potato mash. Spoon the mash into plates and drizzle with

sesame oil. Serve with baked cauliflower.

Per serving: Cal 385; Net Carbs 8g; Fat 35g; Protein 6g

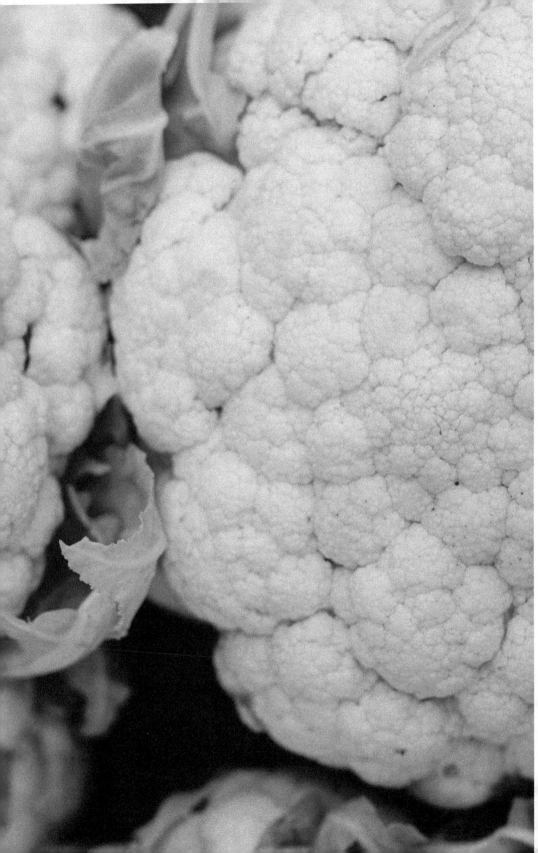

Mushroom Broccoli Faux Risotto

Ingredients for 4 servings

1 cup cremini mushrooms, chopped

4 oz butter

2 garlic cloves, minced

1 red onion, finely chopped

1 head broccoli, grated

1 cup water

¾ cup white wine

Salt and black pepper to taste

1 cup coconut cream

¾ cup grated Parmesan

1 tbsp chopped thyme

Instructions - Total Time: around 25 minutes

Place a pot over medium heat and melt butter. Sauté mushrooms until golden,

5 minutes. Add in garlic and onion and cook for 3

minutes until fragrant and

soft.

Mix in broccoli, water, and half of white wine. Season with salt and pepper

and simmer for 10 minutes. Mix in coconut cream and simmer until most of

the cream evaporates. Turn heat off and stir in Parmesan and thyme. Serve

warm.

Per serving: Cal 520; Net Carbs 12g; Fat 43g; Protein 15g

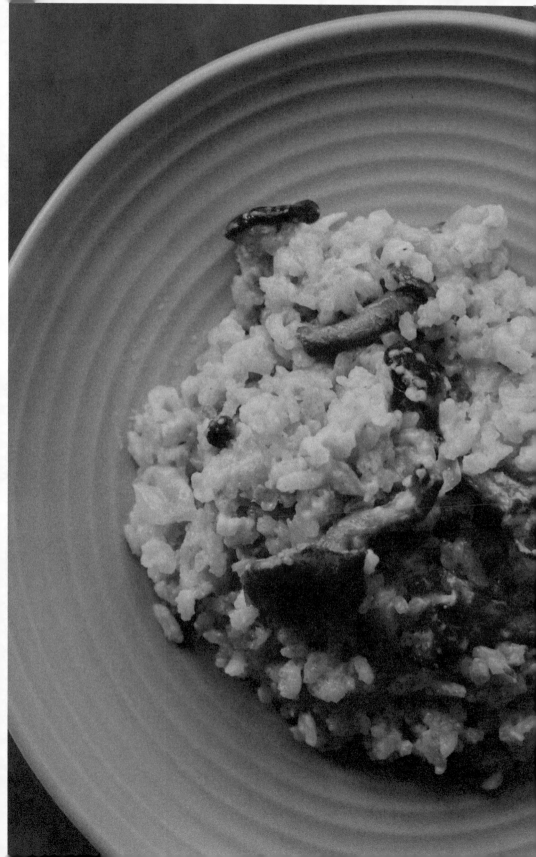

CPSIA information can be obtained
at www.ICGtesting.com
Printed in the USA
LVHW081148110521
687091LV00004B/606

9 781802 328998